Your Next Steps

in

Healthcare
Transformation

J.M. Bohn

Foreword by Audrey D. Kline, PhD

Edited by Rebecca J. Frey, PhD

Copyright © 2011 by J.M. Bohn.
All rights reserved. Printed in the United States of America and all books printed on acid-free paper. Except as permitted under the U.S. Copyright Act of 1976, no part of this publication may be reproduced or distributed in any form or means without written permission of the publisher or authors.

ISBN-13:   978-0-9847641-0-5
ISBN-10:   0984764100

Touchcast Press
Louisville, KY

Library of Congress Control Number: 2011942368
Bibliographic data:

J.M. Bohn
Your Next Steps in Healthcare Transformation   / by J.M. Bohn
p. cm.

1. Healthcare reform. 2. Strategic planning. 3. Change management. 4. Clinical integration. 5. Accountable care. 6. Innovation. 7. Quality improvement. 8. Health information technology.

ISBN: 978-0-9847641-0-5

Contacts-
Copyediting: Rebecca J. Frey, PhD, rebeccafrey@snet.net
Author: J.M. Bohn, joebohn@clinicalhorizons.com

About the Author

J.M. Bohn, MBA, is founder of Clinical Horizons, Inc., focusing on communications, planning, and research efforts related to transformation and innovation in the healthcare industry. Joe holds an MBA from the University of Louisville with a focus on healthcare and economic studies. Bohn has a diverse background that includes five years in the healthcare industry, 10 years in the defense industry, and has operated in the fields of strategic planning, program management, business development, marketing, secondary research, government affairs, and finance along with co-authorship projects on articles, white papers and books.

ACKNOWLEDGEMENTS

The inspiration for this book came from a number of places. We all walk a different path in life and are dealt a different set of circumstances that can shape our existence and path. There are two groups who were most important over the last few years of my life and career that I wish to thank.

First is the nurses, physicians, healthcare executives, and ancillary professionals I've had the pleasure of working for and with during the past five years of my career. Their time and efforts helped educate me on the many nuances of our nation's healthcare system, and made an indelible mark that improved my understanding of the world of healthcare.

Specifically I wish to thank the following healthcare industry professionals for their review and critique of this book prior to publication. Dr. Bruce Flareau, President of BayCare Physician Partners and Executive Vice President of BayCare Health System; Carla Swindle, VP of Clinical Informatics with The Methodist Hospital System in Houston, TX; Sunil Prasad, Director of Enterprise Data Management with MedAssurant, Inc. (www.medassurant.com);

and Marcy Stoots, VP of Optimization and Clinical Adoption for the Healthcare Clinical Informatics Group (www.thehcigroup.com).

Second, I wish to thank the pastors whom I had the pleasure of hearing speak periodically over the past two years. Their messages about life and treating others with honor and respect helped impress the need to make a positive impact upon those around me in society.

PREFACE

Today's healthcare environment is riddled with ever-expanding complexities and challenges that have led to the need for reform. The demographic landscape is changing with the aging of the baby boomers and the coming of age of Generation X and Generation Y, each having its respective cultural, healthcare, and socioeconomic needs. Tackling complex enterprise-level challenges in the healthcare system of the United States is a necessity for organizations to advance to the next level of performance and improve the delivery of healthcare services.

Your Next Steps in Healthcare Transformation is a short book about some important initiatives that represent steps along the path in strategic management of healthcare organizations in their respective cultures and circumstances. This is a new work that is not intended to be all-encompassing, but one that does cover the key initiatives of embracing change; improving quality; managing processes; setting direction; the importance of technology; and innovation.

Purpose of the Book

Your Next Steps has an inspirational and motivational focus. It succinctly covers some important topics being addressed by healthcare organizations and helps readers understand the ever-changing industry as healthcare service delivery enters an era of greater accountability. Important issues addressed include clinical integration, accountable care, drivers of innovation in healthcare, commercial insurance markets, consumer focus, health information technology, local economic impact of healthcare programs, performance measurement, and the general healthcare paradigm shift underway.

Your Next Steps provides 21 original illustrations to help you visualize and understand the various topics presented. As a supplement to Chapter 5, Appendix A provides a select list of resources and initiatives from across the country related to innovation in healthcare. Three personal insights are included to highlight key points throughout the book and emphasize the importance of key issues.

Intended Audience

The intended audience is diverse. *Your Next Steps* can serve as an introduction to key issues being addressed industry-wide for the general public; for interested readers outside the healthcare industry; and for students preparing to enter the industry. For those at higher levels of management or many years of employment in healthcare, the book can serve as a concise overview of several critical initiatives with the potential to generate new ideas and strategic thinking to support plans for future actions.

J.M. Bohn, MBA
October 24, 2011

Table of Contents

Foreword
A New Beginning

In today's politically charged and challenging business environment, healthcare is one of the most important topics under discussion in the United States. The maturing of the baby boomers has had a profound impact on the nation's economy as well as impacting the various industries in which the "Boomers" work and play.

With the plethora of new policies, books, and white papers offering a variety of perspectives on reform efforts in healthcare, *Your Next Steps in Healthcare Transformation* gives us a fresh and concise perspective on key future issues. It focuses on core operational initiatives that are critical not only for healthcare organizations but also for businesses across other industries that need to understand some of the challenges facing the healthcare industry and how they are being addressed.

To move America forward, innovation is needed for success; this need is a central topic in the book. As we advance and work to improve the quality of care delivery, understanding the intricacies and relationships of health outcomes to the economic benefits they will bring to our communities is critically important.

Your Next Steps in Healthcare Transformation provides an overview of many technical issues for its readers. Bohn provides a concise, well-written guide that offers an excellent and comprehensive summary of several key areas for anyone interested in the future of healthcare, from industry professionals to students.

The enormous economic and social impact of the healthcare industry demands that all of us become more knowledgeable about our healthcare system and what we can do to engage in the movement to improve it. This book is a great tool for doing just that.

Audrey D. Kline, PhD
Associate Dean
College of Business
University of Louisville

Chapter 1. Introduction

We are all experiencing tremendous changes in society that are affecting our lives today and that will affect the lives of future generations to come. Improving the health of Americans and our nation's care delivery system has never been more important. Physicians, nurses, educators, policy makers, researchers, employers, and consumers have realized the need for change. This recognition has led to calls for a fundamental restructuring of the United States' (U.S.) healthcare system. An industry rich in tradition focused on improving the quality of life for all patients is in the midst of a transformation that will alter the quality, availability, and affordability of care in North America for years to come.

A movement to meet the challenges ahead is under way.

So how will it all unfold?

It's an ongoing process of improvement that began with the Institute of Medicine's (IOM) 1999 release of *To Err Is Human* that brought to light many factors contributing to the frequent occurrence of medical errors.[1] Numerous reports and studies have been published since then, along with many changes made to improve the system. It's an unfolding that is taking place across the continuum of medical care as the industry works to provide the best quality of care possible.

An Environment in Transition

Generations

Patients in need of care face a financial crisis associated with the rising cost of care. This crisis is amplified by the financial challenges involved in administering healthcare services. The two segments of the general population shouldering the majority of these rising costs is the post-World War II baby boomer generation and Generation X. The oldest members of the baby boomer generation, comprising people born after 1945, reached retirement age in 2010. As a result, the nation's Medicare and Medicaid services confront the challenges of financing the care of what is the single largest segment of the U.S. population. The Medicare Trust Fund's May 2011 Annual Report[2] indicated that the projected growth in funds needed for hospital insurance and supplemental medical insurance as a percentage of gross domestic product (GDP) will steadily rise from its current 3.5+% in 2011 to more than 6% by the year 2050. These projections take into account the expected effects of changes in federal healthcare-related programs in the 2010 Patient Protection and Affordable Care Act (ACA). The projections did not, however, account for the lingering economic recession faced not only by the United States but also globally. From the perspective of patients, caregivers, and physicians alike, the baby boomer generation has a longer life expectancy than past generations and faces many challenges in planning for the future-- of which only a few include:

- ♦ Paying for healthcare on fixed incomes following retirement;

- ♦ Planning for long term and assisted living care needs;

- ♦ Understanding the complex changes affecting Medicare and Medicaid health plans;

- ♦ Evaluating the spectrum of traditional and integrative healthcare services.

The next generation, the so-called Generation X, also faces a number of challenges. This generation, comprising persons born between the mid-1960s and the late 1970s, presently ranges in age from their 30s to early 50s as of 2011. As the baby boomers are entering retirement, Generation X confronts its own set of challenges:

- Continued rising health plan costs;

- Fewer practicing primary care physicians, which causes problems with access to primary care when relocating or changing health plans;

- Fewer services covered by the plans;

- Need for added flexibility with the care they seek (e.g. increased use of retail clinics and services from integrative or alternative medicine practices).

Commercial Insurance Markets

For many Americans today commercial insurance for individuals and families is a top priority, given the rise in healthcare costs. A 2011 report by the Kaiser Family Foundation provided historical statistics for the rise in cost for single and family insurance coverage. The cost of premiums for single coverage rose 8% while premiums for family coverage rose 9%––a substantial increase over the 3% increase borne by consumers in 2009-2010.[3]

A major initiative under the ACA is the future establishment of health insurance exchanges in each state. These new exchanges are intended to increase accessibility to insurance coverage for individuals and small employers in the United States, starting in 2014. A significant problem exists with the United States having 49.9 million Americans (16.3% of the U.S. population) uninsured in 2010.[4] As the health insurance exchange initiative moves forward, it must address the challenge of defining essential health benefits. The Department of Health and Human Services asked the IOM for recommendations in resolving this issue due to its medical, political, and socioeconomic implications.[5] These are only a few of the changes to come in the insurance market. The complexity of the market will continue to be an issue for consumers, provider organizations, and employers for years to come.

While proponents of "big government" and the creation and expansion of federal insurance plans and interventions have helped to accelerate the enactment of reforms, there are also those who take the opposite position. Like President Ronald Reagan, there are those who believe in the free market and the liberties of the individual, and who may choose alternative vehicles to address the complex issues of financing and paying for healthcare goods and services. The debate is certain to continue as the nation moves forward with changing the system of healthcare delivery from its past operations to new models for the future.

Other Implications

Technological changes will continue to have a significant impact in the future along with the transition of care delivery models to new structures. In addition new models of care delivery have emerged that include:

♦ Establishment of clinically integrated networks (e.g. formal networks between physicians and hospitals focused on achieving economies of scale in care delivery and joint contracting with insurers to increase the quality and coordination of patient care[6]);

♦ Start of public and private payer accountable care organizations that focus on improving accountability, performance measurement, and payment reforms in collaborations among physicians, hospitals and other providers that focus on population health management;[7]

♦ Continued adoption and recognition of patient-centered medical homes;

♦ Opening of retail primary care and urgent care clinics over the last several years.

The first three of these models place physicians in leadership to assume ultimate accountability for the quality of care delivered by the organization. In addition they focus on improving financial and health outcomes performance and reporting of the care delivery system.

Another area of importance is the nation's mental health services. Mental health disorders, illnesses, and physical factors affecting mental health can be an internal byproduct of the stressors of the world we live in. Psychiatric services are critical to meeting the healthcare needs of American citizens. A few of the many factors, disorders, and illnesses dealt with daily are identified in Figure 1.

Figure 1. Spectrum of Mental Health Impact Issues

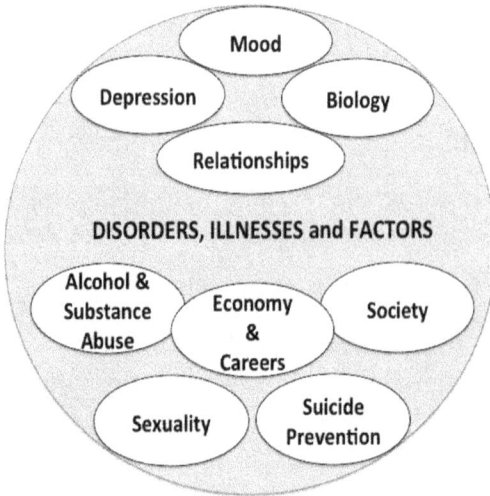

These issues can affect people across all generations and at different times in life. As healthcare reform moves forward, the need to integrate mental health services with other traditional forms of healthcare services continues to grow in importance.

A Movement Under Way

In 2010–2011 the healthcare industry embarked upon a transition from the volume-driven care delivery system of the past–the managed care era that characterized the U.S. healthcare system since the 1980s––to one focused on quality of care; a reward system based on performance and improvement in health outcomes at the population level; and reductions in the cost of care. Figure 2 illustrates this transition.

Figure 2. Healthcare Paradigm Shift

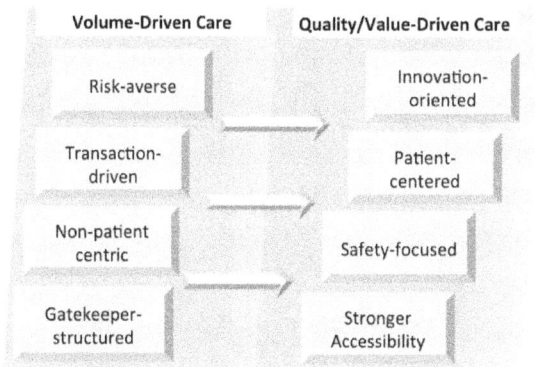

A secondary movement began when this shift started over a decade ago. The managed care model had dominated the industry through the 1980s and 90s, but people recognized that innovation in the way we manage, finance, and deliver care was needed. As pilot projects and other efforts were started in the private and public sectors, observers saw that new incentives and forms of compensation for the delivery of care were also necessary. This recognition brought about the beginning of pay-for-performance models, clinical integration programs, and the dawn of the era of accountable care.

As the Centers for Medicare and Medicaid Services (CMS) established policies for new Medicare accountable care organizations in 2011, they introduced a new set of strategic goals that have been shaped by national healthcare policy initiatives during the past decade. These goals are called the *Three Part Aim.*[8]

Figure 3. Three Part Aim

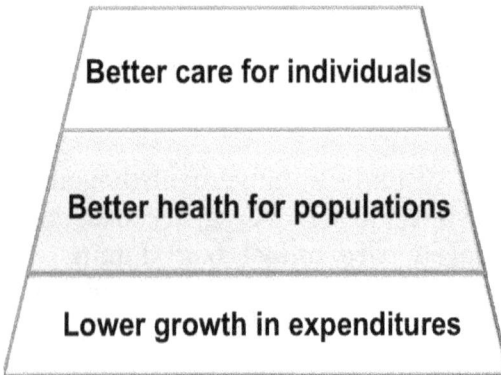

In addition to the *Three Part Aim,* the Department of Health and Human Services established *Six National Priorities* for improving the quality of healthcare in America in 2011. Figure 4 illustrates these priorities. Each is tied to a goal with measures to evaluate effectiveness.[9]

Figure 4. Six National Priorities

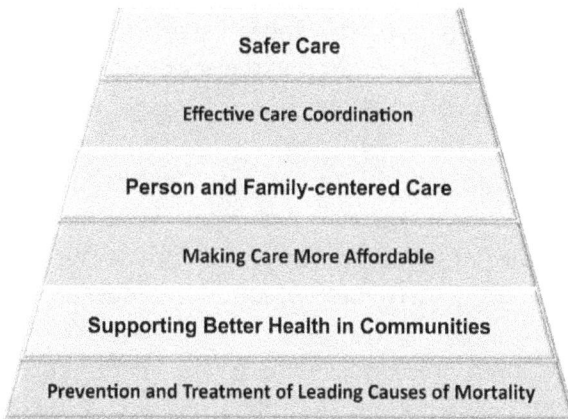

The Department of Health and Human Services website[10] shows the progress that has been made in terms of new programs launched, grants awarded by state, and information on changes in the law that are affecting individuals and businesses alike in regard to efforts to focus on these national priorities. Change was needed and it's occurring. All changes can be related to each of the levels in the focus of the *Three Part Aim* and the *National Priorities*. Some changes will involve trials and pilot projects. Then the industry will evaluate the results and move forward with those that provide the best opportunities to improve the care we deliver.

After noting the aims and priorities, it should be said that while progress is being made, the political debate over the value, necessity, and extensiveness of recent enacted reforms continues. There are many stakeholders impacted by these sweeping reforms, and none more important than the employers across America. Within the employers' sector, one important subgroup is that of the owners of small businesses.

Small businesses are the catalyst of American ingenuity and move our country forward across all industry sectors. Small business owners have faced escalating costs of health insurance for employees for the last several years; today many of them cannot afford to provide individual or family insurance coverage. Companies are seeking alternatives or deciding not to offer health insurance coverage. Herein lies part of the genesis point of plans enacted to establish the state health insurance exchanges starting in 2014––to bring new options for coverage to this vital group of American businesses.

Recognizing this complex set of challenges that exists in the landscape of care delivery today, we must ask who is accountable for the quality of care delivered in the future?

While patients and consumers are responsible for their own health, physicians are the leaders of care delivery who are ultimately accountable for ensuring the quality of patient care. Physicians stand at the forefront of leadership in patient care, clinical integration programs, accountable care organizations, and patient-centered medical homes. In our twenty-first century healthcare system, people should also understand that collaboration in leadership to deliver optimum quality of care and stewardship for healthcare organizations has become increasingly important. The shared decision making between patients and physicians can be extended within organizations to a collaborative plateau with physicians, nursing leaders, other clinical leaders, and administrators. Figure 5 illustrates the collective of disciplines involved in the leadership of today's healthcare delivery organizations large and small.

Figure 5. Collaborative Leadership

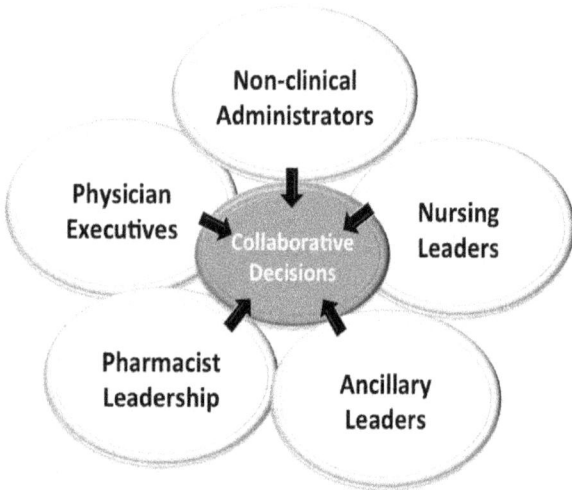

As the industry changes, relationships will be shaped by redefined boundaries that create new roles. Clinical integration programs are one example of an increasingly important initiative for healthcare services delivery across geographic regions. They underscore the need for collaboration, physician leadership, adoption of health information technology, and a continuous focus on improving health outcomes for communities across the nation.

Your Next Steps

This introductory chapter describes a few of the issues affecting contemporary healthcare. It sets the context for discussing *Your Next Steps in Healthcare Transformation* in the chapters that follow. Each step represents a major foundational initiative (not all inclusive) for healthcare organizations and stakeholders that can be taken sequentially or non-sequentially by all participants in our nation's healthcare system.

What are the initiatives to be discussed?

The following chapters provide details for the initiatives outlined in Figure 6.

Figure 6. Your Next Steps for Healthcare Transformation

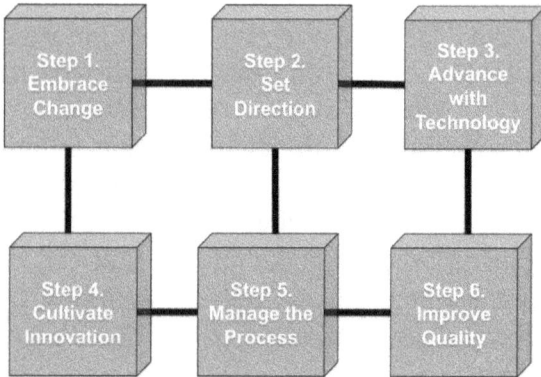

Step 1. Embrace Change

Step 2. Set Direction

Step 3. Advance with Technology

Step 4. Cultivate Innovation

Step 5. Manage the Process

Step 6. Improve Quality

These six initiatives cover a broad range of requirements needed to identify opportunities and take action to improve healthcare services and products in today's challenging economic climate. Physicians, nurses, ancillary and administrative professionals, and healthcare leaders are often engaged in all these initiatives depending on their organization's situation. Such other functional areas as finance and accounting, pastoral care, information services, health information management, risk management, legal, managed care contracting, and others have tremendous importance to the operation of a healthcare system; however, the focus of the following chapters is on these six initiatives. Today clinical and administrative professionals are contributing to positive changes in our nation's healthcare system and to the growth of our nation's healthcare workforce.

Our Opportunity

The chance to take that quantum leap is here. The seeds to reform healthcare have been planted and several organizations have been leading the way for years. It's time to change our nation's healthcare system for the benefit of generations to come.

** If you could improve one element of healthcare in America over the next two years what would it be and how would you do it?

What is offered in this work is not a comprehensive plan but an introductory overview of these six types of initiatives to help stimulate creative thinking and planning activities.

Chapter 5 will cover topics in the field of innovation: Appendix A provides a list (not comprehensive) of select resources focused on the field of innovation in healthcare.

This book should be considered a tool to supplement strategy with illustrated concepts that can advance one's level of knowledge in key areas and spur creativity for you and your team. It is a work to help educate those not directly engaged in transforming our nation's healthcare system.

Perhaps serving as a starting point for some and a bridge to complementary ideas for others that will help you and your organization in charting the course for *Your Next Steps in Healthcare Transformation*.

"The journey of a thousand miles must begin with a single step."

Lao Tzu (570-490 B.C.)
Chinese philosopher

1 Institute of Medicine, Committee on Quality of Health Care in America. Executive Summary. In: *To Err Is Human.* Washington, DC: National Academies Press, 2000, pp. 1-5.

2 Medicare Board of Trustees. Overview. In: *2011 Annual Report of the Boards of Trustees of the Federal Hospital Insurance and Federal Supplementary Medical Insurance Trust Funds*, p. 17. Accessed online September 21, 2011 at https://www.cms.gov/ReportsTrustFunds/downloads/tr 2011.pdf.

3 Kaiser Family Foundation and Health Education & Research Trust. Section One: Cost of Health Insurance. In: *Employer Health Benefits, 2011 Annual Survey*. Menlo Park, CA: Henry J. Kaiser Foundation, 2011. pp. 10-24. Accessed online October1, 2011 at http://ehbs.kff.org/?page=charts&id=2&sn=16&p=1.

4 DeNavas-Walt, Carmen, Bernadette D. Proctor, and Jessica C. Smith, U.S. Census Bureau, Current Population Reports, P60-239. Health Insurance Coverage in the United States. In: *Income, Poverty, and Health Insurance Coverage in the United States: 2010*, Washington, DC: U.S. Government Printing Office, 2011, p. 22. Accessed online October 1, 2011 at http://www.census.gov/prod/2011pubs/p60-239.pdf.

5 Iglehart JK. Defining Essential Health Benefits — The View from the IOM Committee. *New England Journal of Medicine* 365 (October 20, 2011):1461–1463.

6 Flareau B, Yale K, Bohn JM, Konschak C. Leadership. In: *Clinical Integration: A Roadmap to Accountable Care*. Virginia Beach, VA: Convurgent Publishing, 2011, p. 68.

7 Fisher ES, McClellan MB, Bertko J, et. al. Fostering accountable health care: moving forward in Medicare. *Health Aff (Millwood)*. 2009;28(2):w219-w231; Flareau B, Yale K, Bohn JM, Konschak C. Glossary and Acronyms. In: *Clinical Integration: A Roadmap to Accountable Care*. Virginia Beach, VA: Convurgent Publishing, 2011, p. 325.

---

[8] Federal Register vol. 76, no. 67. April 7, 2011. I.(C) Overview and Intent of Medicare Shared Savings Program, p. 19533.

[9] Department of Health and Human Services. *Report to Congress: National Strategy for Quality Improvement in Health Care.* March 2011. Accessed online October 2, 2011 at http://www.healthcare.gov/law/resources/reports/quality03212011a.html.

[10] Department of Health and Human Services webpage on status of health law changes. Accessed September 28, 2011 at http://www.healthcare.gov/law.

Chapter 2. Embrace Change

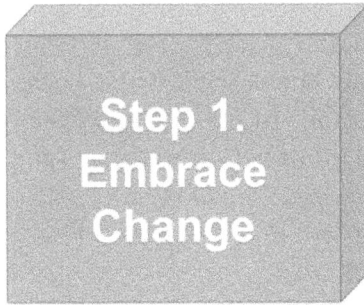

The U.S. healthcare system is undergoing changes that affect all of us across society as patients, consumers, healthcare workforce, suppliers, and employers. These changes drive financial, clinical, socioeconomic, and political decisions that impact healthcare organizations large and small. What are some of the factors driving these systemic changes? Four key factors are as follows:

1. **Complexity**- The U.S. healthcare system is a complex adaptive system with many interconnected elements that can present new challenges and produce new efficiencies, but also result in unintended adverse consequences for patient care or patient relations. The intricacies of the system and the cause

and effect that each element has on other elements can complicate the reengineering of the processes involved. Complexity, when not understood can lead to chaos, but when resources are dedicated to assess interrelationships throughout networks and organizations, actions to advance efforts can be identified and negative effects can be minimized.

2. **Workforce Transition-** Each generation produces new physicians, nurses, ancillary professionals, and others with new ideas, understandings, and abilities to improve organizations and the patient care services they deliver. As the dynamics of healthcare service delivery have changed, how we prepare medical, nursing, and other healthcare students for their chosen fields of practice has improved and will continue to evolve. In addition the changes involved in the role of nursing professionals advancement into leadership positions continues across the industry in clinical operations, administration, information services, education, risk management, and consulting among other areas.

3. **Economic Transition**- Because the nation as a whole is affected by global economic trends, the financial health of U.S. healthcare organizations is affected by the crises and daily cycles of global financial markets.

4. **Demographics**- One of the most profound and often remarked demographic issues driving change in our nation's healthcare system is that of the baby boomer generation. The financing of services needed to care for the members of this generation in the latter stages of their lives with both public- and private-sector resources is and will continue to be a key issue requiring systemic changes for decades to come.

In addition to these factors driving systemic change in the healthcare provider sector, as noted in Chapter 1, the public and private payer health insurance market is also experiencing a paradigm shift. Significant changes are taking place across the commercial payer segment of the industry through the ACA. Three major changes affecting this payer segment include:

- Elimination of preexisting conditions as a reason for denying coverage;

- Requiring 80-85% of premiums to be spent on health services and healthcare quality improvement;

- Planning for the market's transition to health insurance exchanges for individuals and small employers.

As the healthcare industry adjusts to these changes and others involving the contractual dynamics and relationships among payers, providers, and consumers, managing change will be a necessity.

Addressing Needs

Where do we go today that we don't see a need for change? Are there still situations where there is resistance?

Nurses, physicians, and ancillary staff members must deal daily with operational changes as workflow is redesigned in their practices, hospitals, and other care settings. Changes required in accommodating new technologies, clinical guidelines, new safety standards, and ways to measure efficiency and effectiveness are all being implemented at a rapid pace.

One key to understanding the need for change is recognition. Once people recognize the need, they can then be stimulated by a sense of urgency and motivated to take the necessary actions. One of the most influential change management experts in the last two decades is John Kotter who formulated an eight-step approach to managing change in any organization.[11] The implementation of changes such changes as electronic health record (EHR) implementations; joint ventures between hospitals and physician practices; the transition of the health insurance industry to state-level health insurance exchanges; and other enterprise-level programs will require the application of Kotter's methodology.

Figure 7 is an illustrated adaptation of Kotter's eight-step approach.

Figure 7. Kotter's 8-step Approach

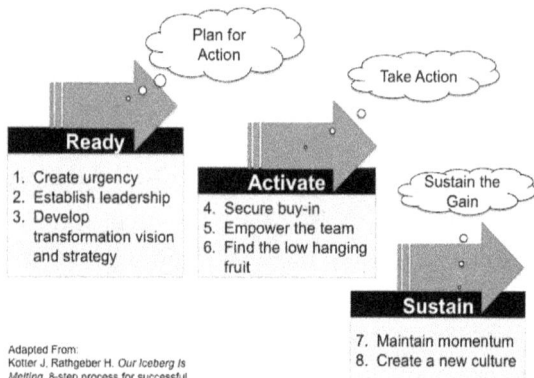

Plan for
Action

Take Action

Ready
1. Create urgency
2. Establish leadership
3. Develop transformation vision and strategy

Activate
4. Secure buy-in
5. Empower the team
6. Find the low hanging fruit

Sustain the Gain

Sustain
7. Maintain momentum
8. Create a new culture

Adapted From:
Kotter J. Rathgeber H. *Our Iceberg Is Melting*. 8-step process for successful change. Pages 130-131.

One can see the practical benefits of Kotter's methodology in its three stages. Regardless of the issue, event, or transition under way, these eight steps allow us to peel back the layers of the onion; find the root cause of a problem or the need for change; and stimulate transformational action that brings teams, constituents, organizations and other entities to a new plateau where they can better achieve the goals they establish whether small or large.

Managing the Change Factors

The four key factors driving systemic change listed above all have one feature in common. They are part of the impetus affecting the transformation of healthcare in our nation. While debate continues in regard to the multi-generational impact of landmark healthcare reforms passed in recent years, it is clear that change was needed. One thing is certain: there will be more changes in the future.

That said one of the four major factors of systemic change is complexity. Our healthcare system has evolved into one of the most complex business models in existence. As a complex adaptive system, it can be thought of as a network (or multiple networks) within a larger network (e.g. federal, state, and local markets all structured by competing forces to provide healthcare services for various segments of the population). Other issues that affect the system's ability to function adequately and efficiently include:

♦ Organizational culture

♦ Need for patient-centered care

♦ Influence of new technologies

♦ Barriers to progress: fragmentation and decentralization

♦ Focus on evidence-based medicine

♦ Consumer interest in integrative or alternative medicine

♦ Payment model innovation

♦ Care delivery model innovation

♦ New laws for the evolving system

Collectively, such issues as these can increase the magnitude of interconnectivity in the system. Figure 8 illustrates these issues within four quadrants representing the four key factors driving systemic change.

Figure 8. Interconnectivity

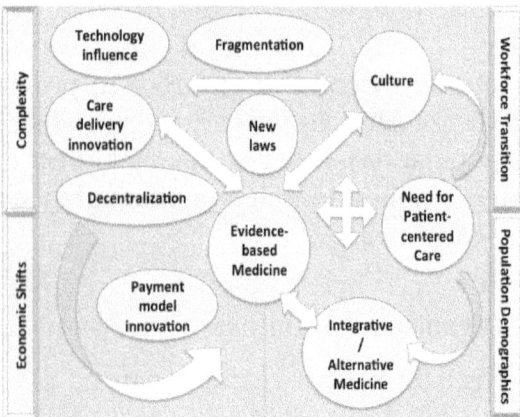

This arrangement of issues presents some of the dynamics and reasons for the complications faced today in our evolving health system. The issues within the four quadrants could be arrayed in multiple configurations. Decentralization and fragmentation can be byproducts of the system's evolution over the last century, but these characteristics have imposed burdens on the efficiency and effectiveness of the U.S. healthcare system. Second, while complexity is one of the four key factors, by its nature it can be a trait of each of the other four quadrants. Finally, each of the nine issues contributes to the broader challenge to remedy systemic problems causing inefficiency, increasing costs, and ineffectiveness passed on to patients, consumers, and other stakeholders.

So how do we manage some of the forthcoming large-scale industry changes?

A few important points to consider when addressing change in your own organization or program include:

♦ Developing and appointing champions to facilitate the adoption of new values and new systems;

- Addressing the various concerns of constituents;

- Recognizing the complexity of the system and actions needed to reduce negative effects on healthcare system performance and patient care outcomes;

- Assessing organizational ability to deal with forthcoming changes regardless of whether they are internally driven or externally generated.

Dealing with change will require addressing constraints but also openness to new possibilities to improve organizations and the way we deliver care. Accept and embrace the challenges and we can change the world of healthcare. Leave the processes and patterns of the past behind and welcome the new age of healthcare in America with a focus on improving it for the next generation.

Chapter 2: Takeaways

✓ Recognize the importance of Kotter's methodology for managing change.

✓ Understand the four factors causing changes in the U.S. healthcare system.

✓ Identify the nine issues that impact the system's ability to function adequately and efficiently.

✓ Illustrate the interconnections among the factors causing systemic change and the issues rooted in the dynamics of complexity.

"No one is demanding that we like the change, but the sooner we see it and set out to become an irreplaceable linchpin, the faster the pain will fade, as we get down to the work that needs to be (and now can be) done."[12]

Seth Godin (1960-)
Author, innovator, and entrepreneur

---

[11] Kotter J, Rathgeber H. The Eight Step Process of Successful Change. In: *Our Iceberg Is Melting*. New York, NY: St. Martin's Press, 2005, pp. 130–131.

[12] Godin S. *The forever recession (and the coming revolution)*. Seth's Blog September 30, 2011. Accessed online October 2, 2011 at http://sethgodin.typepad.com/.

Chapter 3. Set Direction

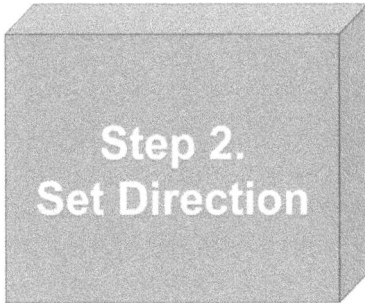

Direction setting in today's world is critical for all organizations; and aligning direction with your mission and vision is essential. Alignment is necessary to ensure successful efforts in business. Without it, inefficiencies arise and chaos may result. There are, however, many factors to consider when setting direction for your organization.

What are some of these factors?

♦ Organizational culture

♦ Value system

♦ Ties to stakeholders

♦ Customer connections

♦ Industry dynamics

When we look at what is happening in healthcare today, and especially here in the United States we can see the need to realign goals. The system lacked alignment for several decades as a result of its complexities, challenges, barriers and other factors. However, lessons were learned and factored into future strategies and plans that helped bring about the paradigm shift that is underway. Reforms such as the growth of clinically integrated networks, patient-centered medical homes, and launching accountable care organizations, are at the forefront of the industry realignment that is embodied by the shift from a culture driven by volume of care delivered to one focused on quality and value.

Mission and Vision

The mission of healthcare is ultimately to care for and improve the heath of the patients served. If we loose sight of this mission for even a moment and fail to maintain it at the forefront of our daily work, we risk losing sight of the purpose and meaning of our work. Every physician, nurse, clinician, information technology leader and staff, and administrative personnel working in healthcare knows this and it is ingrained in the culture of contemporary healthcare.

Insight #1: Mission

The mission of healthcare. Its essence is simple, but achieving excellence in its delivery is complex: the calling to serve as healers and to help those in need.

For those with non-clinical experience it can be tremendously valuable to experience the *heart of the mission* of patient-centered care first hand. Seeing the power of those who care for the sick and their ability to cope, compartmentalize, diagnose, and deal with daily pressures is critical to understand the mission. It can provide the "*ah ha*" moment needed to grasp the mission of healthcare delivery at a deeper level beyond administrative operations.

Each organization's mission should include a statement of purpose for its existence, its part in making the U.S. healthcare system incrementally. Next after the mission is the leader's vision. In order for that vision to take hold and serve as a beacon for the future, this vision must be shared with others throughout the organization. Peter Senge said it best,

Ultimately, leaders intent on building shared visions must be willing to continually share their personal visions.[13]

A key point here is continual sharing. Repetition reinforces the intent and shows commitment on behalf of the leader's part. Figure 9 illustrates that both mission and vision should lead to development of the organization's goals. Ensuring integration of these core planning elements is part of solidifying each organization's strategy framework.

Figure 9. Strategic Framework Alignment

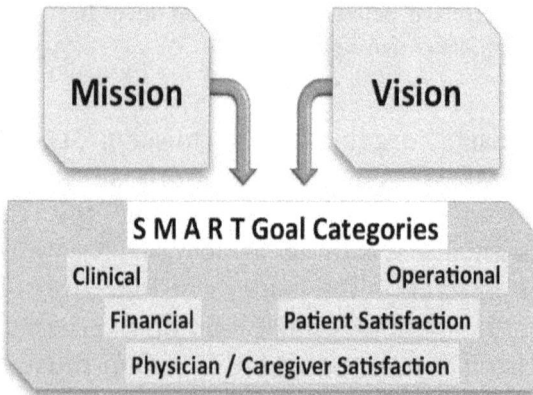

Mission → Vision

S M A R T Goal Categories

Clinical   Operational

Financial   Patient Satisfaction

Physician / Caregiver Satisfaction

SMART Goals

Can a healthcare organization establish meaningful goals without a shared vision?

When this linkage is not present within the strategic framework, incongruence and lack of connection can surface and lead to inefficiency or loss of direction. The U.S. healthcare system is realizing greater benefits from reducing barriers, allowing better evaluation of the effectiveness of processes and systems that operate across settings--which makes the integration of these strategic elements even more important. In the area of transition in care delivery models, the nation is moving toward more clinically integrated networks that adopt this linkage of strategic elements to measure efficiency, quality of care, and reductions in medical errors more effectively.

As healthcare organizations transform their cultures and structures, they must have goals that provide meaningful assessments of progress. Figure 9 illustrated five categories of goals. For organizations to capture the value they are delivering, their goals should offer insight into their community economic impact and health outcomes for the communities and patient populations they serve. Having measures to assess the five areas of clinical, financial, operational, physician/caregiver satisfaction, and most importantly patient satisfaction will allow the organization to understand how its actions are affecting their patients, communities and progress toward its shared and common vision.

For goals to be meaningful, the SMART analogy can serve as a foundation for ensuring practical assessment. Figure 10 illustrates the SMART approach to goal-setting.

Figure 10. SMART Goal-setting

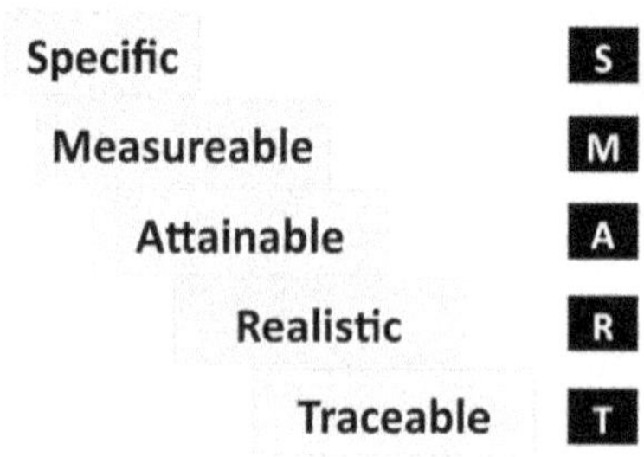

Specific	S
Measureable	M
Attainable	A
Realistic	R
Traceable	T

What program or initiative are you working on and what are its goals?

Whether your goals are clinical, operational, or administrative, you can look at them and determine whether they possess the SMART characteristics. The importance of goals and measuring our performance as an element of *Your Next Steps* will be discussed further in Chapter 7.

In examining your personal goals, do they align with the goals of the organization you work for?

When so much of our time in life is spent in our profession, true alignment between the personal and organizational sets of goals leads to opportunities to succeed and to capitalize on one's intrinsic motivation. In America, more than in any other country in the world, we have freedom of choice; we have the power to change.

The opportunity to assess direction as individuals and improve the health of our communities has never been greater. To set organizations on a better path is part of the essence of healthcare transformation. To determine the goals for providing better care for all segments of our population, regardless of demographic/socioeconomic backgrounds, we can work to measure and achieve systemic improvement one patient at a time.

Chapter 3: Takeaways

✓ Alignment of mission, vision and goals is a critical part of each organization's strategic framework.

✓ It is important for leaders to share their visions as emphasized by Senge.

✓ Having SMART goals supports alignment and can help provide meaningful insights to progress and impact.

"What you get by achieving your goals is not as important as what you become by achieving your goals."

Hilary *"Zig" Ziglar (1926-)*
American author and
motivational speaker

---

[13] Senge P. Chapter 11. Shared Vision. *In: The Fifth Discipline. The Art and Practice of the Learning Organization.* New York, NY: Doubleday Currency Publishing, 1990, p. 215.

Chapter 4. Advance with Technology

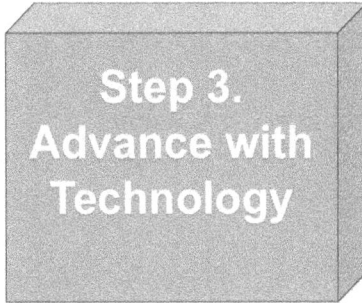

Much of contemporary society's progress is being driven by global transformation through technology. For much of the twentieth century, many industries here and abroad were established and run by the standards of the industrial revolution of the nineteenth century. The twenty-first century, however, is the Internet age, in which Web-based technology is transforming the way we live, work, communicate, and play around the globe.

It's impossible to cover all the changes related to technology occurring throughout healthcare and the larger society in this chapter. Most communities and organizations, however, are reengineering their processes, pathways, and cultures with technological advances being made on a daily basis. The iPad, satellite communications, new laser scopes for surgical procedures, smaller and faster computers and cell phones, and the embedding of social media as part of our global culture are a few examples of advancements that have organizations throughout society adopting new tools more rapidly than ever before in history.

But can we keep pace with the rate of change?

Accepting change as discussed in Chapter 2 is critical to success; but recognizing boundaries and the fact that setbacks will occur is also very important. There are a multitude of technological advances that could be described that are affecting care delivery at the patient, community and population level. Lets look at a few, with a focus on the field of health information technology (HIT), which is transforming the landscape of healthcare services.

Elements of Transition

The transformation underway is altered daily by the launch of new tools and applications, many of which are bringing about paradigm shifts in the way healthcare is delivered. Just as we are seeing the shrinking of newspapers and other forms of print media in society, so too is this move to digital media and communications taking hold in the world of healthcare.

The introduction of electronic medical records (EMR) started in the late 1960s but their adoption was extremely slow for several decades. Over the years, however, studies of the benefits of EMRs were done and the healthcare community realized the need to adopt this form of record keeping to meet the challenges of the twenty-first century. EMRs are part of the global development of HIT that will enable other transformational changes in the industry. In addition, a major change will occur in 2013 with the conversion of medical coding in the United States to the International Classifications of Diseases Tenth Revision (ICD-10). This change will expand the coding of discases, medical terminology and diagnoses exponentially. While much of the industrialized world is already using ICD-10, all participants in the U.S. healthcare system will make this change simultaneously.

Figure 11 provides an illustration of several (but not all) key technological advancements in the HIT arena.

Figure 11. A Foundation for Growth

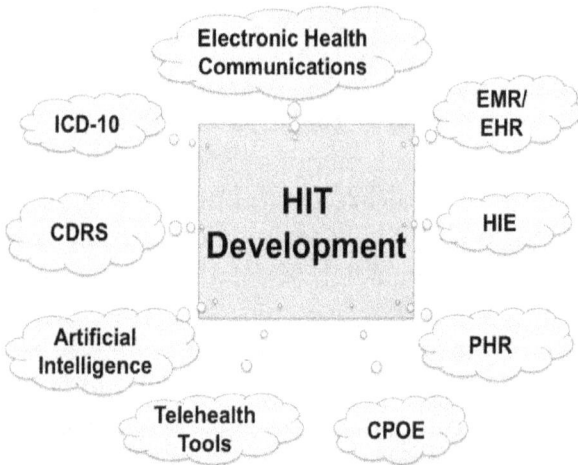

Each technology has significance in its part of the spectrum of new tools and applications in development and use today. As many of these tools were put to use across healthcare settings throughout the industry over the past decade, the Department for Health and Human Services created the Office of the National Coordinator for Health Information Technology to provide strategic national oversight.[14] This organization has served as a focal point for the rollout of several new programs that are accelerating the advancement of technological capabilities through funding of new demonstrations, incentives, and HIT implementation support programs.

How do organizations deal with the challenge of prioritizing the development, financing and adoption of so many new tools?

Meeting this challenge requires leaders knowledgeable of and experienced in critical decision-making. An understanding of the risks involved, the benefits to be derived, and the impact on other systems and operations helps to set the right course. Underlying each of these technology areas is the rapidly growing need for clinical data warehouses to serve as repositories for the massive amounts of data collected. These warehouses are needed for analyzing and providing the right data at the right time to support clinical decision-making. Much of HIT in development today serves to improve capabilities and efficiency for those on the frontline of care and to streamline operations.

Setting priorities and planning for adoption is where the skill and experience of physicians, nurses and other healthcare leaders come into play. Without their knowledge of the complexity of clinical workflow, and the ramifications of making changes to various systems as well as the impact on patient care services, the opportunity to *hit the mark* and achieve the greatest benefit is lost.

Insight #2: Leadership in HIT Adoption

The ability of physicians, nurses and ancillary leaders to drive collaborative initiatives across clinical disciplines and settings is essential. Ensuring effective communication through champions at the early stage of enterprise-level HIT implementations can produce large gains across clinical domains. It can ensure that organizational and cultural barriers are removed, risk of failure is reduced, that *priorities are understood*, and that plans are communicated effectively.

Having addressed EMRs/EHRs, clinical data warehousing, and ICD-10, two other foundational enablers to address are electronic health communications and artificial intelligence.

Electronic Health Communications-

The advent of the Internet and social media spawned new capabilities for industry with digital communications for consumers, healthcare workers, and patients alike. Such sites as Facebook, PatientsLikeMe, Sermo, CaringBridge, LinkedIn, and others are all being used in various ways to help improve knowledge sharing. The Internet connects patients with other patients and allows them to access healthcare information pertinent to their situation. Connecting physicians to other physicians for sharing of best practices and connecting physicians to patients through secure communication channels that meet health data privacy requirements is all being enabled rapidly. In light of the growing use of these new tools over the last decade, many organizations have now incorporated policies for the use of social media websites to govern employees' use of them for the benefit of their organization, communities, and patients. One such example is the Centers for Disease Control and Prevention (CDC) that provides detailed guidelines for its employees regarding communication strategies, clearance for posting information, and best practices for using Facebook.[15]

The use of mobile applications and smartphones has created new access points to enhance physician-to-patient and physician-to-physician knowledge sharing opportunities. These technologies have also increased communication on public health issues along with integrating diagnostic applications that use radio frequency transmitters and sensor technologies to provide physicians with real-time health monitoring data to physicians on a patient's health status. This field of technology is likely to see rapid growth in future years.

Artificial Intelligence-

Research and development of applications using artificial intelligence (AI) has accelerated considerably for HIT, medical devices, other aspects of healthcare, and biomedical technologies. Such industries as aerospace and defense have demonstrated some of the most notable applications of AI, as seen in unattended sensor technologies, unattended aerial and ground vehicles, among others.

Some advances in healthcare to date are in the fields of robotics and clinical decision support tools. The continued development of artificial intelligence within many tools helps improve predictability and reactions or responses of technologies to different situations and processes where they are used. Key challenges that continue to be addressed with artificial intelligence are in the areas of knowledge management, problem solving, response planning, and learned behavioral responses––all of which require further development of new applications in the care delivered to patients across settings and multiple types of care givers.

The Future Is Here

The impact of these new tools, systems, applications, and ways of communicating will be felt for generations. We are moving into an era in which clinically integrated organizations are the norm, HIT brings new capabilities and improves decision making, and geographic competition changes with the transformation of care delivery models. As the technology and communication infrastructure is strengthened throughout rural and urban America, *Smart Cities* (e.g. communities with advanced information technology infrastructures, wireless capabilities, and advanced energy grid systems to support economic and social development in their region for multiple industries and consumers alike) will continue to come of age with continued improvements in mobile applications and associated infrastructure and the increased deployment of sensor technologies. With a more comprehensive approach to future healthcare knowledge management the equation is simplified:

BETTER INFORMATION
+IMPROVED CARE DELIVERY
=
BETTER POPULATION HEALTH

The economic impact of these advances in healthcare systems is significant. In the near term there are cost burdens related to the implementation of foundational technologies, systems that enable health information exchange (HIE), creation of data warehouses, establishment of telehealth capabilities, and a continued push toward establishing a national health information network (NHIN). In the long term, benefits will increase as efficiency gains continue to emerge and the industry moves past its learning curve and implementation expenditures; and as the next generation of healthcare workers enters the workforce with new ideas and familiarity with technologies and tools. The economic impact and benefits to population health outcomes will need continual assessment to validate the impact of these developments on the baby boomers, Generation X, and other demographic segments of society.

Unintended consequences are certain to occur with HIT as it evolves and efforts to increase our vigilance in monitoring relationships between patient safety and implementation of new HIT will continue to grow as the industry moves forward.[16] However, it is important to acknowledge these issues and work to mitigate negative impacts as part of the ongoing process of transforming the healthcare system in the United States and around the globe.

Clinical integration is leading the move to the era of accountable care. Working to *"increase the interdependence and cooperation among physicians with the intention of controlling cost and improving quality of care delivered"*[17] is one of the keys to success for clinical integration programs. These efforts establish a new structural foundation with technological enablers for physicians, nurses and others in clinical and administrative operations to better measure the quality of care delivered.

As part of *Your Next Steps* in healthcare transformation the new tools, systems, applications and other technologies on the horizon should continue to be evaluated and adopted when needed to help achieve the *Six National Priorities* for the U.S. healthcare system.

Chapter 4: Takeaways

- ✓ EMR adoption continues to accelerate.

- ✓ There are many elements on the landscape of HIT development.

- ✓ The expanding use of electronic health communications is certain to continue in the future.

- ✓ Recognize the importance of exploring opportunities with artificial intelligence.

- ✓ *Smart Cities* will continue to mature along the path with communications and technology infrastructure.

"Design must reflect the practical and aesthetic in business but above all. . . good design must primarily serve people."

Thomas J. Watson (1874–1956)
Founder and president of IBM

[14] Office of the National Coordinator for Health Information Technology website. Accessed October 2, 2011 at http://healthit.hhs.gov.

[15] Center for Disease Control and Prevention. *Social Media Guidelines and Best Practices.* Updated January 3, 2011. Accessed online October 2, 2011 at http://www.cdc.gov/SocialMedia/Tools/guidelines/pdf/FacebookGuidelines.pdf.

[16] Institute of Medicine, Committee on Patient Safety and Health Information Technology. Summary In: *Health IT and Patient Safety: Building Safer Systems for Better Care.* Washington, DC: The National Academies Press, 2012 (pre-publication copy), pp. S3–S6.

[17] Department of Justice and Federal Trade Commission. Enforcement policy on physician network joint ventures. Statement #8, Section 8A. Accessed online October 2, 2011, at http://www.ftc.gov/bc/healthcare/industryguide/policy/statement8.htm.

56-Your Next Steps

Chapter 5. Cultivate Innovation

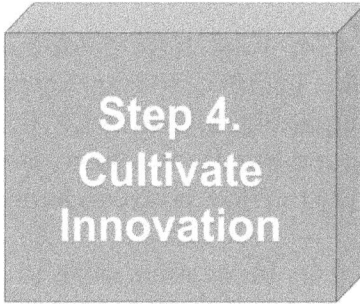

Step 4. Cultivate Innovation

The dawn of a new age in healthcare is upon us. The industry is being supported by innovations that were beyond the scope of our technical capabilities just 10 years ago. New ideas are being generated every day, and they are making the world a better place to live with new opportunities to save lives. It's how we improve what the previous generation was able to deliver through the advances in technology, improvement in processes, and new ways of thinking.

Innovation is a key to every model of transformation for every industry; without it we become stagnant and progress is stifled. With it, we continue to advance as a society. Some innovations are incremental, however, while others are paradigm-shifting.

Step 4 in *Your Next Steps* to ensure success in healthcare transformation is about cultivating innovation. Evaluating big ideas and small ones alike, brings the opportunity to effect positive change.

What does innovation mean to you and for our twenty-first century healthcare system?

Society and healthcare are changing at a rapid pace. Innovations are serving as enablers of needed change. As technology is advancing, consumers, patients, and stakeholders of the healthcare system are communicating and working with new tools. The industrial age has given way to the age of the Internet with Web 3.0 right around the corner. While the Internet is still evolving, it is certain to involve new levels of intelligence built into the future Web-based tools and sites that will occupy cyberspace.

Innovative ideas are needed to advance therapies, therapeutic delivery systems, care delivery models, and HIT systems for today's U.S. healthcare system and future generations of patients and stakeholders. Innovations foster competition and enable us to improve quality. They will help meet emergent patient needs that results in stronger quality of care for the baby boomers, Generation X and Generation Y alike.

Certainly there are several issues that are driving this requirement for continuous innovation. Figure 12 identifies a few of them:

Figure 12. Issues Driving the Need for Innovations in Healthcare

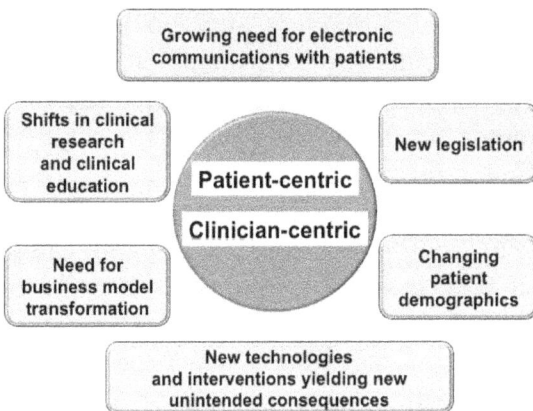

There are two core elements to Figure 12: the central focus on patient-centric and clinician-centric solutions and six issues underlying the need for innovation to advance the quality of healthcare services and products.

First, when new innovations are conceptualized, the patient should be at the center of the concern underlying the idea. As the IOM noted in their landmark 2001 report, *Crossing the Quality Chasm: A New Health System for the 21st Century*, patient-centeredness is one of the six goals for healthcare improvement.[18] Coupled with this aim is the notion of clinician-centric as another major focus for developing innovations that are useable, practical and obtainable solutions for the needs of physicians, caregivers, and ancillary staff to meet current and future challenges in care delivery. One example of clinician-centric innovations is the need that was recognized years ago to expand broadband Internet access to healthcare providers and facilities in rural communities. As many applications are Web-based, communities that did not yet have access were unable to move forward with implementing or adopting many technological advances. Today the industry is closing that gap to the Internet access challenge.

A few keys for effective innovation development in the future of healthcare include balancing:

♦ Effective evaluation of innovation ideas;

♦ Speed in bringing to innovations to market;

♦ Understanding benefits, risks, and rewards;

♦ Potential for both dissemination and diffusion of the innovation;

♦ Determining the potential for positive effects on outcomes, access, quality, and cost of care;

♦ Resonance with patient-centeredness and clinician-centric foci.

There are many great healthcare organizations across our nation working on innovations to solve current challenges. They are working in public, private, academic, and nonprofit sectors. A few are identified for reference in Appendix A. Within each organization's purpose and business processes is the strong commitment to innovation in its culture and a drive to find opportunities to improve the quality of care in America.

Second are the six issues identified in Figure 12. Each of these issues generates new requirements for people, processes, and systems to improve the quality of care delivered. Lets address two of the six as examples.

New Legislation: The Health Information Technology for Economic and Clinical Health Act (HITECH) and ACA are recent *examples of new legislation* at the federal level. Their enactment established new policies to meet the emerging needs of physicians, hospitals, patients, consumers and other stakeholders in the U.S. healthcare system, and to encourage research for additional innovations. As industry-level requirements for innovation are identified, there is also a need for federal- and state-level legislators to change laws and regulations to allow initiatives to proceed. While the process of developing and enacting new legislation can take months to years, it serves as a mechanism to transform the healthcare system as organizations look beyond the near term for systemic innovations to close the gaps in quality, access, and cost of care.

The Growing Need for Electronic Communication with Patients: Patients in today's world are demanding increased electronic communication with their physicians and clinician care providers. As communication throughout the rest of society has shifted to digital media, there is a growing need for secured electronic patient communications as noted in Chapter 4. Many patients are now highly accustomed to e-mail, chat, texting, and other forms of electronic messaging. As a result many physicians and other care providers have sought new Internet-based technology solutions, social media sites related to healthcare, and other applications to meet patient demands.

Recognizing that these needs exist, how do we manage the growth and spreading of new ideas?

Out of the Box

The growth of new ideas requires a process to bring them forward (think of it as getting them *out of the box*) to cultivate, disseminate and diffuse them. Means of doing this will vary across organizations with some being more complex than others. The passage of the America Invents Act[19] will have a long-term effect on research and development, innovation idea disclosure, dissemination and diffusion of innovations, and many other issues related to changes in patent law.

Organizations will seek or pursue a variety of innovations at various points in their business life cycle. Some innovations have the potential to change the game, such as disruptive innovations as defined by Harvard professor Clayton Christensen while others serve to incrementally improve upon existing products or services. These can be considered sustaining innovation.[20]

So how should an organization to cultivate a continuous flow of new ideas? Especially ideas that may address *unmet needs* and close gaps in the quality, cost and accessibility of healthcare services?

One model is presented in Figure 13. This model depicts four conceptual areas: a) internal network; b) external network; c) whiteboard arena; and d) pipelines.

Figure 13: Cultivating Innovative Ideas

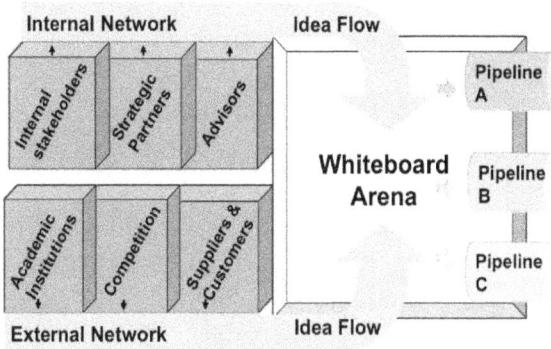

The notion of seeking ideas from both internal and external networks is drawn from the example of Proctor & Gamble's Connect and Develop innovation model that has served as one strategy for their product research and development for several years.[21] The internal networks may include individuals with a contractual relationship to the entity. The external network recruits participants beyond the organization's direct control. As ideas are generated from both types of networks the ideas are funneled into a central planning area that we'll call the *whiteboard arena*. Here is where the initial review, vetting, and filtering of ideas can take place. From this point new ideas can be directed into various pipelines (such as A, B, and C in our model) in which experts in the subject matter of the respective areas channel the ideas for review and further consideration.

This model has been simplified as an instructive example. Academic research institutions, nonprofits, private sector, and public sector organizations engaged in research and innovation will have highly complex models in terms of their organizational structures, laws and governance requirements.

What are some examples of ideas that come from either network in the case of a healthcare services organization?

♦ Opening new service lines to address specific needs of baby boomer patients in the market served;

♦ Creating and offering novel incentives to physicians and caregivers;

♦ New ways to select vendors;

♦ New methods for controlling health service utilization and costs;

♦ New HIT systems to improve clinical outcomes and increase efficiencies in clinical operations;

♦ New communication tools to improve relationships with existing and potential patient populations.

New ideas are generated daily as entities work to improve competitiveness and better serve the populations they care for across the country. In regards to the overall process of innovation development, there are other elements of importance. A few of them include:

♦ The next stage in channeling ideas through a vetting process;

♦ Identifying intellectual property that can be culled from innovation ideas;

♦ Measuring the risk-reward and cost-benefit tradeoffs of each idea.

One key to cultivating new ideas is the participants' level of *commitment*. Models for developing innovations inherently invoke a process that must be prepared for failure. Without openness to failure, the testing and determination of which new concepts, product ideas, business models, or potential service lines have the best chance to improve the quality of care while lowering costs of care may be lost. The need for experimentation may be compromised when a *lack of commitment* exists and opportunities disappear.

Understanding Benefits

Innovation is essential for the growth of organizations. Of course the potential to find the idea that will lead to the next generation iPhone, a new telemedicine service, or a new use for excess facility capacity to increase revenue and care for more patients, is what drives all industry participants to seek new ideas. Changes in payment processes for hospital and physician services, evolving cultural expectations, and the overall structure of the healthcare system continue to push large and small organizations to streamline their activities and search for those ideas that will lead them to a better future.

What are a few of the benefits with innovation planning?

Figure 14 identifies a few benefits to be derived from innovation planning.

Figure 14. Innovation Planning Benefits

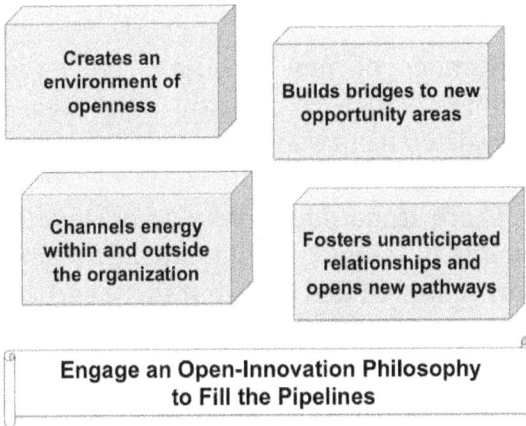

Creates an environment of openness

Builds bridges to new opportunity areas

Channels energy within and outside the organization

Fosters unanticipated relationships and opens new pathways

Engage an Open-Innovation Philosophy to Fill the Pipelines

In addition to these benefits it is important to assess quantitative measures of performance of an organization's efforts in innovation planning and management. Many ratios can be used to evaluate progress. Assessments should be made at such different stages as: a) idea generation, b) review and vetting of new ideas, c) production or operationalizing of the idea, and d) post-market launch. A few examples of assessment include:

♦ Number of ideas generated per business unit vs. cost spent generating those ideas;

♦ Annual funds spent on protection of knowledge and intellectual property derived from the innovation program;

♦ Number of new products or service lines launched annually vs. revenue realized from them.

There is no single way to achieve the benefits in innovation planning. One model is presented in this book but there certainly are many others. Different ratios may be used to evaluate progress or effectiveness between internal and external networks or for different groups based on their industry, environment or situation.

So this is *Step Four*: getting your ideas to the whiteboard arena and taking the risk of sharing them and presenting a different concept. Your ideas may involve changes for people, processes, technologies, or cultures, but as we discussed in Chapter 2: welcome change, and we can change the way we deliver care. If we never try, we will never fail, but we will also never have the chance to succeed. In this critical period for American medicine, it is vitally important to continue *cultivating innovations*.

Chapter 5: Takeaways

✓ Sustaining and disruptive innovations are both important.

✓ Get your ideas to the whiteboard arena.

✓ It's important to always measure the impact and benefits of innovation efforts.

✓ Remember that success cannot come without some possibility of failure.

✓ Capitalize on both your internal and external networks.

✓ Pay attention to generational patient needs in conceptualizing innovations.

"Learning and innovation go hand in hand. The arrogance of success is to think that what you did yesterday will be sufficient for tomorrow."

William G. Pollard, PhD, MA (1911–1989)
Physicist

[18] Institute of Medicine, Committee on Quality of Health Care in America. Patient-centeredness. In: *Crossing the Quality Chasm: A New Health System for the 21st Century*. Washington, DC: National Academies Press, 2001, pp. 48–51.

[19] United States Patent and Trademark Office. America Invents Act. September 16, 2011. Accessed online October 1, 2011 at http://www.uspto.gov/aia_implementation/bills-112hr1249enr.pdf.

[20] Christensen CM, Grossman JH, Hwang J. The Role of Disruptive Technology and Business Model Innovation in Making Products and Services Affordable and Accessible. In: *The Innovator's Prescription. A Disruptive Solution for Health Care.* New York, NY: McGraw-Hill, 2009, pp. 3-6.

[21] Huston L, Sakkab N. Connect and Develop: Inside Procter & Gamble's New Model for Innovation. *Harvard Business Review*, 84 (March 2006):58-66.

Chapter 6. Manage the Process

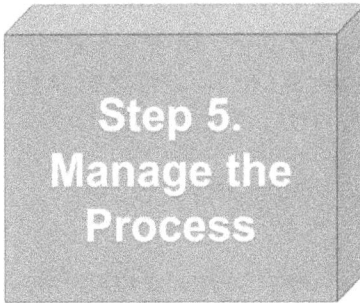

In all facets of business and clinical operations across healthcare settings there are processes, projects and programs to manage. Ensuring that participants and stakeholders understand scope, deadlines, penalties and rewards for completing efforts on time and within budget is crucial in today's deadline driven and budget conscious world.

Step 5: Manage the Process is about the importance of managing all the individual projects that can roll up to programs within large-scale healthcare transformation processes that bring about fundamental change. A healthcare organization's goals for cost control, ensuring quality, and meeting deadlines are a priority for executives, physicians, researchers, and clinicians at all levels. While we discussed the issue of embracing and managing change in Chapter 2, here we consider a few of the strategic and technical elements of managing tasks within a transformation process.

Projects Within the Process

Project management methodologies and tools assist small as well as large organizations (e.g. service providers, physician practices, technology vendors, insurance companies, and others) in assessing progress toward their goals. Efforts can range from development of high-level communications involving one or two individuals, to complex programs for new HIT systems that may involve hundreds to thousands of individuals across multiple settings.

One of the industry standards to manage large-scale efforts in project management is the *Guide to the Project Management Body of Knowledge (PMBOK Guide)*, produced by the Project management Institute (PMI).[22] Figure 15 illustrates three key points for managing the processes to reach intended goals.

Figure 15. Process Management Strategy

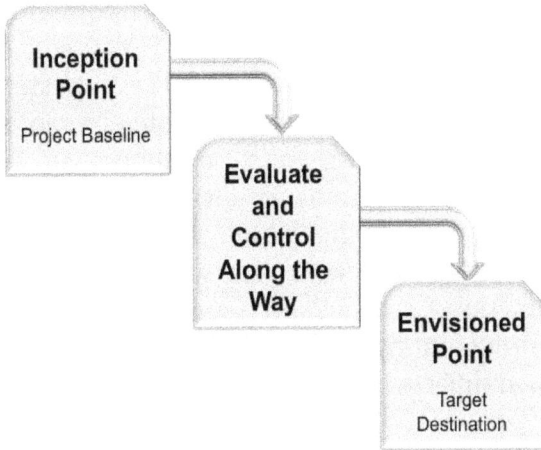

Core steps in managing the process and the projects within it to successful completion are as follows:

↓ *Recognize and document the original baseline or point of inception*

↓ *Evaluate progress along the way*

↓ *Reach the target destination with an implemented project/program*

The PMBOK methodology is important for large projects and programs because it provides the structure to give healthcare executives status reports on quality, expenditures, and schedule performance. When these efforts involve significant resources and personnel extending over months and sometimes years (such as HIT system implementations and care delivery model transformations), the methodology is particularly beneficial. Figure 16 provides a Gantt chart illustration that is not time-scaled but serves as an example of functional tasks to monitor in HIT implementation. While this example is oversimplified, Gantt charts are a highly effective tool for tracking and reporting progress.

Figure 16. Sample Project Gantt Chart

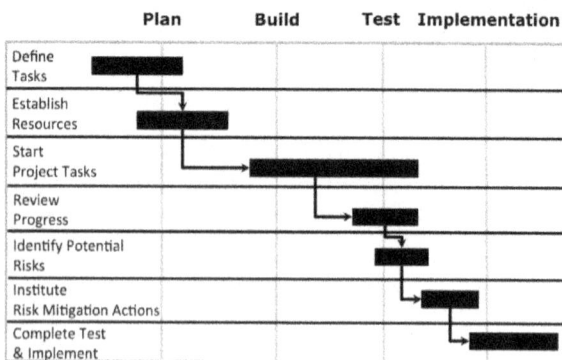

	Plan	Build	Test	Implementation
Define Tasks				
Establish Resources				
Start Project Tasks				
Review Progress				
Identify Potential Risks				
Institute Risk Mitigation Actions				
Complete Test & Implement				

HIT Implementations

How easily can one loose control of the process in an HIT implementation?

Without the right leaders, monitoring mechanisms to mitigate risks, project management staff, and other resources... it can happen easily due to the many challenges with such implementations. For example, EMR implementations, in light of their complexity and invasiveness into so many aspects of a healthcare organization's workflow, can benefit tremendously from application of project management tools that instill a degree of trust and due diligence in the oversight process.

Using the right methods and tools assists' managers in controlling risk, limits scope creep, and increases opportunities to control costs in HIT implementations.

Care Delivery Model Implementations

With efforts growing across the country to implement clinically integrated networks, accountable care organizations, and patient-centered medical homes in the primary and specialty care practices, managing the process for these culturally redefining initiatives will be essential to their success. PMBOK methodology is equally applicable to these transformations. They provide ways to assess progress, status reporting on scope changes, and evaluations of an organization's cultural changes under the new care delivery model.

As the landscape of healthcare organizations, their services, and HIT and medical device vendors changes in the coming decade, the methods used and how we manage the transformations may be affected by:

CULTURAL SHIFTS

POPULATION DEMOGRAPHICS

SPEED OF CHANGE

NEW TECHNOLOGIES

Think about these factors. First, our global community is shrinking. Cultures are colliding; philosophies and ways of living are changing as we encounter the new forms of interconnectivity that link us all. Second, the aging of the baby boomer population requires new projects to be managed and planned.

While tools and technologies may change, there are certain attributes that are critical to the success of the process with any HIT implementation or transition to a new care delivery model. A list of these attributes appears in Table 1 below.

Table 1. Success Attributes

Attribute
Determine scope
Establish goals
Set and manage schedules
Quality control and integration
Team building
Resource management
Identify and mitigate risks
Control costs

In transformation efforts there will be some degree of activity that can be controlled and other activities that cannot. Regardless of the size and scope of a project it is important to remember the significance of *managing the process* to maintain progress for the benefit of our healthcare system in the twenty-first century.

Chapter 6: Takeaways

✓ Have a project strategy in place at the beginning of each project/program.

✓ Make sure that every project is marked by the attributes of success.

✓ Recognize factors that may affect future projects.

"Effective leadership is putting first things first. Effective management is discipline, carrying it out."

Stephen Covey, DRE, MBA (1932–)
American author and consultant

---

[22] *Guide to the Project Management Body of Knowledge (PMBOK Guide).* Newtown Square, PA: Project Management Institute, 2008.

Chapter 7. Improve Quality

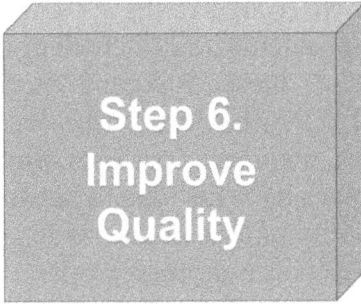

What will a better healthcare system look like 10 years from now?

How different will it be from where we are today?

IMPROVED COORDINATION

FEWER MEDICAL ERRORS

GREATER SYSTEMIC CONNECTIVITY

IMPROVED EFFICIENCY

REDUCED INCIDENCE OF CHRONIC DISEASE

GREATER COST CONTROL

Improving our national system of healthcare delivery in the United States is critical as we recognize the systemic nature of our problems and challenges. The visibility of these systemic issues has increased over the last three decades as consumers, taxpayers, patients, physicians, and clinicians have become better informed on the quality of care delivered in America. Web-based tools have increased:

♦ Knowledge-sharing;

♦ Insights into transparency of the quality of health services;

♦ Performance of vendor products and systems;

♦ Awareness of medical errors and health outcomes for all population segments and demographic groups.

In line with these insights, U.S. healthcare organizations are moving away from the volume-driven transaction-focused way of delivering care of the past. In turn they are transitioning toward models of care delivery focused on patient-centeredness, improving communications, and achieving better outcomes with lower cost of care.

Trends

In 2001 the IOM identified four underlying factors associated with inadequate care in the U.S. healthcare system. These are illustrated in Figure 17.[23]

Figure 17. Causes of Inadequate Care (IOM, 2001)

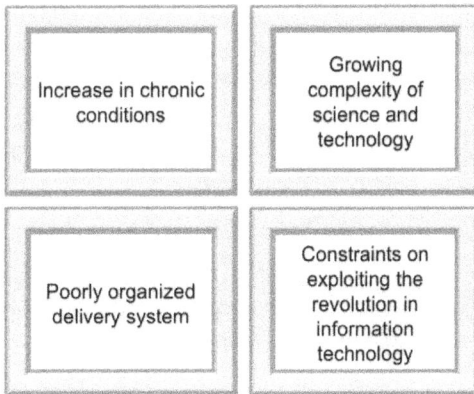

Increase in chronic conditions	Growing complexity of science and technology
Poorly organized delivery system	Constraints on exploiting the revolution in information technology

As a nation, we have made great progress in addressing some of these underlying causes. We have, however, experienced different degrees of progress with mitigating each of these causes over the past 10 years.

Chronic Conditions: Type 2 diabetes is an example of a chronic condition that was known to be on the rise in 2001. In 2002 there were an estimated 18.2 million diagnosed and undiagnosed cases in the United States.[24]   The most recent data indicates that there are 25.8 million cases of diagnosed and undiagnosed cases of diabetes in the United States; this trend is expected to continue.[25]

Delivery System Organization: In the past, delivery systems were relatively fragmented and decentralized. Today this problem is being resolved as the cottage industry continues to shrink, mergers and consolidations increase in number, and expansion of clinical integration programs and accountable care organizations reduce the healthcare industry's degree of fragmentation and decentralization.

Complexity of Science and Technology: The nation's healthcare system has grown in complexity since 2001. The complexity of science has helped drive this increasing complexity in healthcare. The systems and processes for which we access and pay for care have grown as a result of research findings and technological advancements that have supported the growth of evidence-based medicine. While having solved some systemic problems this has also created new challenges and served as evidence of the increasing complexity of science in its impact on healthcare. Technology itself has also continued to increase in its complexity since 2001. A number of examples of new trends and developments in health information technology were addressed in Chapter 4, many of which emerged or accelerated in development during the last decade. Technologies have assisted in dealing with many challenges; however, as demand for interoperability, faster communications, and new tools increases, additional layers of complexity in systems will continue to emerge.

Constraints Exploiting the Revolution in HIT- A number of constraints existed at the time of the IOM's report that hindered the industry's ability to advance the use of HIT. Great progress, however, has been made with incentive programs, pilot projects, validating the benefits of different systems and tools, and more widespread adoption of HIT led by key healthcare organizations across the country.

These trends were already visible in 2001, and as the industry witnessed throughout the past decade, the importance of finding solutions to each one only continues to grow. New organizations emerged focusing on the unique challenges posed by each of these trends, but more work remains to reduce future impact of these causes of inadequate care. Given that these causes of inadequate care are reinforced by such others, as complications in financing healthcare services and physician or hospital compensation for delivery of care; and administering the safety net infrastructure, we must evaluate performance and progress from both the clinical and economic perspectives.

How do we know when we are truly making progress?

How do we evaluate progress for both individual-level improvement in outcomes and community-level improvement in outcomes and economic impact?

A key trend is the increased emphasis on measuring performance. Such new programs as CMS's Meaningful Use of EHRs started in Phase I (2010) with a set of quality measures that will expand in Phase

II and III of the program. In addition CMS launched the eRx Incentive Program in 2009 along with the Medicare Shared Savings Program (starting in 2012) both of which are performance-driven based on evaluations against specified performance measures and benchmarks. As these programs are focused on the Medicare beneficiary population, valuable insights will be gained on the system's performance in meeting the healthcare service and product needs of the baby boomer population in the coming decades. Such other performance measurements as the Healthcare Effectiveness Data and Information Set (HEDIS) serve as key reporting requirements for private payer health plans. Harmonizing these different performance measures is becoming a major necessity across the industry. It will become more feasible as such technological capabilities as those discussed throughout Chapter 5 come to maturity.

Healthcare organizations across the United States will continue to emphasize quantifiable performance measures to better assess progress in improving health outcomes and the effects on local economies.

Local Economic Impact

Chapter 1 noted the long-term projections for the growing percentage of GDP that will be required to cover the costs of healthcare in the coming decades. In order to reduce these projections, healthcare organizations across the country have been engaged in both vertical and horizontal mergers that affect the supply of healthcare workers and their ability to meet the demand for services from communities across the country. New programs with a focus on improving health outcomes for targeted segments of the population continue to emerge along with these organizational changes, reforms, and technological advances, as we move toward more clinically integrated networks of care.

Measuring the economic impact in each community in terms of local efforts in new healthcare service programs and market competition is one way to confirm the value derived from program and systemic changes. Some of the effects to examine include:[26]

- **Employers**: labor efficiencies resulting from streamlined operations and workforce education;

- **Employers and Consumers**: increased absenteeism and labor costs resulting from employee healthcare issues; costs of health plans to all constituents;

- **Healthcare Organizations**: impact of technological changes on workforce efficiency (near- and long-term) and consequent cost reduction in providing healthcare services;

- **Population Disease Management**: effectiveness of disease- or disorder-focused programs' on reducing costs of care for targeted subpopulations in each community.

Tracking our progress on these issues and many others will convey the economic benefits for consumers and employers in specific communities. Coupling measures of these issues with the performance measurements of outcomes provides a complementary and more complete view for healthcare leaders, community leaders, employers and the general public of the comprehensive value gained from the implementation of new healthcare programs.

Performance Measurement

The *Three Part Aim* (Figure 3) and the *Six National Priorities* (Figure 4) discussed in the Introduction provide a new foundation for future strategy and actions to be aligned with directives on the national level. These aims and priorities evolved over the past decade through system redesign along with recognition of the need for changes in leadership, education, and the structure of care delivery models. But the need for more meaningful assessment also required further work to support key decisions and enable healthcare executives to set a better direction.

Performance measurement refers to assessing progress and determining the path forward when goals are reached as well as when they are not reached. It involves applying quality management methodologies and tools such as:

♦ **Six Sigma:** quality management doctrine that was developed by Motorola in 1980s; first applied in manufacturing industry and has spread to be used across many industries globally with a focus on making statistically significant improvement in processes;

♦ **Lean:** methodology that focuses on preserving value and eliminating waste; originally conceived by Toyota in the 1990s;

♦ **PDCA (plan-do-check-act):** quality improvement methodology used to work toward continuous improvement of processes developed by Dr. W. Edward Deming.

These methodologies and tools are used to analyze and reengineer clinical and administrative processes to eliminate waste, improve efficiency, and reduce cost. Making goals measureable is a prerequisite for setting an organization's direction.

Avedis Donabedian, MD, who is widely considered the father of healthcare quality management, gave us a framework of three dimensions—structure, process, and outcomes—to assess healthcare quality.[27] Figure 18 illustrates Donabedian's three dimensions, which still embody much of what is done in healthcare today.

Figure 18. Donabedian's Quality Framework

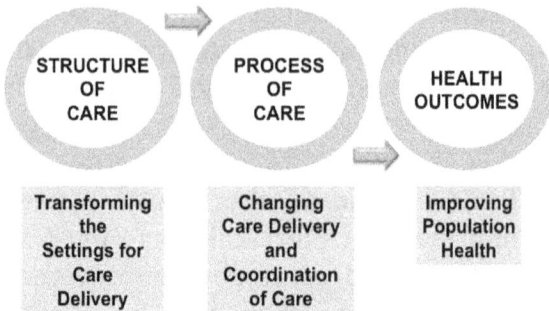

Applying Donabedian's framework to quality assessment can lead to a range of questions regarding each dimension.

STRUCTURE

Is the setting right for our patients?

PROCESS

How do we measure our clinical work?
Is it effective?
Is the workflow efficient?

OUTCOME

What is our patient's quality of life?
Are we seeing improvements in our ability to treat specific conditions?

These are just a few of the possible questions that prompt the development of quantitative measures and setting SMART goals. Such questions help organizations determine the impact on each of the three dimensions of healthcare quality.

Several organizations are working to refine quality measures as the landscape of care delivery is being transformed. Many different quality measures have been developed and approved by the National Quality Forum, one of the industry's leading endorsers of quality measures. Some of the issues encouraging refinement of measures include:

♦ Changes in care delivery models;

♦ New collaborative processes;

♦ Technologies to measure and evaluate impacts across populations;

♦ The future transition to ICD-10.

Each of these issues among others will bring about meaningful changes in how we evaluate and measure the quality of care delivered in our twenty-first century healthcare system. Figure 19 illustrates another perspective on the evolution of performance measurement during the past decade.

Figure 19. Changes in Performance Measures

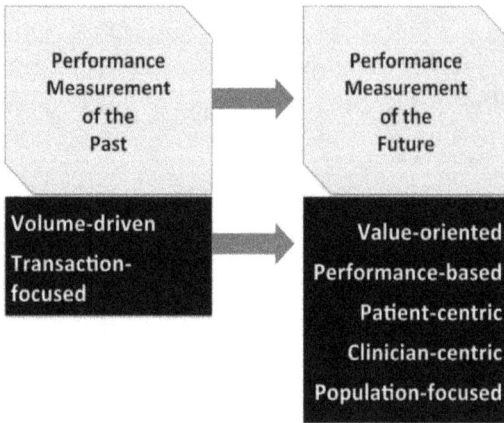

As this transition continues in the coming years, one thing is certain: changes in how we assess performance will improve understanding of the quality of care delivered for physicians, clinicians, and the patients they serve.

Reporting to Leadership

Leaders of healthcare organizations need regular assessments of their measures of success. Monitoring an organization's status in meeting performance expectations in delivering the best patient care possible requires data and information necessary for critical decision-making. Therefore defining appropriate measures of success appropriately is critical.

What are some of the keys to defining an organization's measures of success?

♦ Engage the stakeholders;

♦ Set SMART goals that link to the vision, mission, and the organization's or program's priorities;

♦ Measure the right things at the right times;

♦ Make sure that measures are valid, reliable and understandable;

♦ Analyze results accurately.

Insight #3: Measures of Success

Enterprise-level transformations require the identification and development of "measures of success" in order to evaluate the present and future effects of the new program. Meaningful quality metrics have become increasingly important to physicians, nursing leaders, and all ancillary professionals on the front line of care across care settings.

Such programs as CMS's Meaningful Use of EHRs, Physician Quality Reporting System and the eRx Incentive Program provide performance assessments, insights, and status on progress for measuring the quality of care delivered.

Scorecards are a critical tool used for reporting progress on programs, projects and operations to leadership. They can be used to present results of both quantitative and qualitative measures of interest to leadership. A few common items to consider when structuring a scorecard are identified in Figure 20.

Figure 20. Common Scorecard Elements

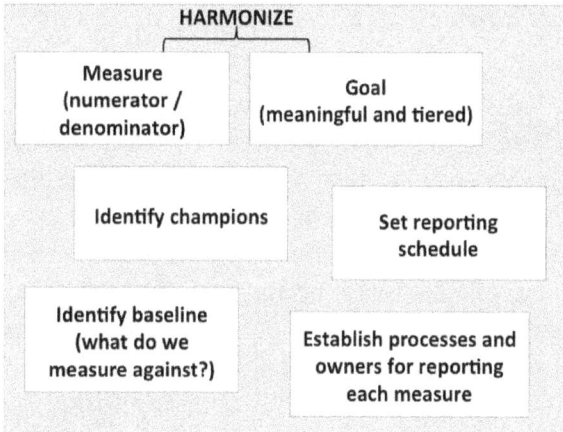

Many healthcare organizations will select measures of success based on existing programs that include measures that are regularly reported on regularly to external parties. These include CMS value-based purchasing programs, clinical integration programs, CMS Meaningful Use of EHRs, patient-centered medical homes, and accountable care organizations.

Major initiatives are taking shape across the industry to improve quality throughout healthcare. Automation and continued implementation and adoption of EHRs will continue to bring new opportunities to improve quality reporting as manual efforts are phased out and give way to real-time assessments at the level of the individual patient, care setting, and population.

Given the importance and promise of EHRs, a significant number of studies were conducted in the last decade regarding their impact and effects on quality of care. One element of these systems that was focused on was computerized physician order entry (CPOE). Two key studies of interest was one published by Ross Koppel and colleagues in 2005 that identified 22 types of medical errors involving a CPOE system[28] and a second published in 2006 and 2007 by Joan Ash, Dean Sittig and colleagues that identified nine types of unintended consequences related use of CPOE.[29] The intent here is not to address the types of medical errors or the unintended consequences in detail, but to raise awareness of the need to identify and track these issues in quality scorecards for physicians, healthcare executives and other stakeholders to have greater insight to their impact on processes, people, and the population level quality of care delivered.

As we reduce the complexities, refine the culture, and work toward more patient-centered care operations in all healthcare organizations, new initiatives will emerge that require continued assessment of performance across structure, process, and outcomes.

Chapter 7: Takeaways

✓ Remember the three dimensions of the Donabedian quality framework.

✓ Understand the history and status of the causes of inadequate care.

✓ Work toward securing characteristics of the future health system.

✓ When reporting to leadership, give meaningful performance assessments on regulatory and culture change objectives.

"Quality is everyone's responsibility."

W. Edwards Deming, PhD, MS (1900–1993)
Consultant, author and professor

---

23 Institute of Medicine, Committee on Quality of Health Care in America. Underlying Reasons for Inadequate Quality of Care. In: *Crossing the Quality Chasm: A New Health System for the 21st Century*. Washington, DC: National Academies Press, 2001, pp. 25-33.

24 Centers for Disease Control and Prevention. 2003 National Diabetes Fact Sheet. Accessed online October 1,

2011 at
http://www.cdc.gov/diabetes/pubs/estimates.htm.

[25] American Diabetes Association. Data from the 2011 National Diabetes Fact Sheet (released Jan. 26, 2011). Accessed online October 2, 2011 at http://www.diabetes.org/diabetes-basics/diabetes-statistics/.

[26] Teitelbaum JB and Wilensky SE. Health economics in a health policy context. In: *Essentials of Health Policy and Law*. Sudbury, MA: Jones and Bartlett Publishers, 2007, pp. 64-71.

[27] Stanford University. (June 2007). Closing the Quality Gap: A Critical Analysis of Quality Improvement Strategies. *AHRQ Technical Review Number 9. Chapter 5. Conceptual Frameworks and Their Application to Evaluating Care Coordination Interventions*, Section 5b. Methodological Approach, Model 2: Donabedian's Quality Framework.
Accessed online October 2, 2011 at: http://www.ncbi.nlm.nih.gov/bookshelf/br.fcgi?book=hstechrev&part=A25445.

[28] Koppel R, Metlay JP, Cohen A, et al. Role of Computerized Physician Order Entry Systems in Facilitating Medication Errors. *JAMA*, 2005;293(1):1197-1203.

[29] Campbell EM, Sittig DF, Ash JS, Guappone KP, Dykstra RH. Types of unintended consequences related to computerized provider order entry. *J Am Med Inform Assoc*. 2006;13(5):547-56; Ash JS, Sittig DF, Poon EG, et al. The extent and importance of unintended consequences related to computerized provider order entry. *J Am Med Infom Assoc*. 2007;14(4):415-423.

Chapter 8. The Path Ahead

Momentum is increasing in the transformation of the way healthcare will be delivered to future generations in the United States. To continue progress, however, we must "*take action.*" Those who are in leadership must empower those around them. Those who are on the front lines of care must serve with intention and respect. Administrators must study areas that are foreign to them to better understand the roles and responsibilities of those they support. In order to "*sustain the gains*" we need a plan as well as innovation.

For healthcare service innovators and researchers, continue to bring your ideas forward. Consider ideas that come from outside the box and outside your comfort zone; evaluate with a critical eye, but never be afraid of failure.

Know that there will be hurdles to cross and at times the path may not be clear--but together we can change the system, making it a patient and family-centered system--one that doesn't fail:

OUR PATIENTS

OUR FAMILIES

OUR COMMUNITIES

A system that continuously refines itself, learns from its mistakes, and recognizes that failure at times is required to achieve greatness. The system depends on the continued implementation of new HIT from which new solutions will emerge. It's just the beginning. When we achieve nationwide interconnectivity for every doctor and every hospital in America then new goals will emerge to continue improving the system.

Looking Forward

As a collective, for those striving to help others and lead organizations, the path may be similar. The system has been fragmented and decentralized but we are making strides to improve it.

What is the path to improving the system?

Your Next Steps has identified six initiatives that are broad in scope, but each can help advance the system of healthcare in our nation. Figure 21 summarizes four elements important for the path ahead. Without change we remain stagnant––thus recognition of the need to act is essential. Sometimes failure comes from trying to *"get things right."*

Figure 21. Focus Going Forward

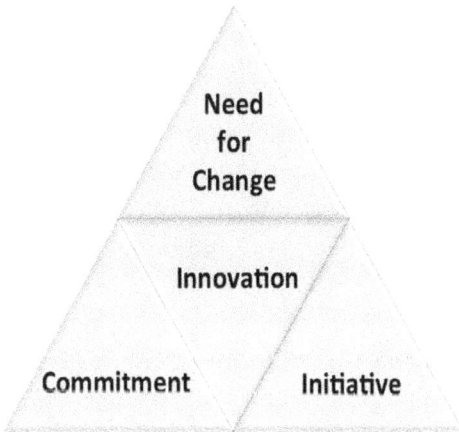

These four elements serve as a summary of some key points from the earlier chapters. Each one is critical in continuing to improve the quality, access and cost of healthcare in the United States.

1. **Need to Change**: Chapter 2 described the importance of welcoming change. Before we do so, however, we must recognize it and follow up with action to champion a cause or make a difference. The four factors involved in systemic change can serve as stimuli to launch efforts or champion a cause. Writing and publishing the IOM's landmark reports (*To Err Is Human* and *Crossing the Quality Chasm*) required the work of healthcare leaders, industry champions, researchers, and policy makers to improve the quality, access and cost of care in our healthcare system. Lessons learned from the managed care era and problems caused by the cottage industry structure of primary and specialty care have also led to recognizing the need to remedy the challenges of industry fragmentation and decentralization.

2. **Innovation**: As discussed in Chapter 5, at the heart of the U.S. healthcare system's renaissance is a passion for innovation. While clinical research in this country has been driven by the search for innovations for decades, the importance of defining and launching new models for care delivery and

payment or reimbursement has gained momentum in the last decade. With the escalation in the cost of care, the aging of the baby boomer generation, and the need to deliver higher quality with improved efficiency, such organizations as the Center for Medicare and Medicaid Innovation are emerging with the goal of stimulating further innovation. Advancing these models and a national agenda to encourage creativity will require many positive character traits: but two prominent success factors are commitment and initiative.

3. **Commitment**: Without commitment as described in Chapter 3, progress is slow and in many cases cannot be made at all. Individuals and organizations with commitment will be engaged in their tasks, supportive of those joining their cause, and dedicated to delivering results.

4. **Initiative**: To succeed in bringing new devices or other inventions to market. The desire and perseverance to finish a project (such as an engineer who works tirelessly to fix a system design flaw) is critical to successfully complete a mission.

A key feature in the transformation of healthcare in America is the transition from a volume-driven system to one measured by quality and value. As Porter and Teisberg noted in *Redefining Healthcare*,

> The right objective for health care is to increase the value for patients, which is the quality of patients outcomes relative to the dollars expended.[30]

As we look ahead, we should recognize the need to change and encourage industry participants to develop new innovations, compete, and to deliver services based on value and quality. The nation's healthcare system will continue to build its clinically integrated capacity to support future generations. On the path ahead we can see the necessity of clinical integration and the future of accountable care; it's a place in which the landscape of competition for future healthcare services and products is retooled for the benefit of patients, consumers and other stakeholders in the U.S. healthcare system. Today we are on the brink of great changes that will lead to substantial improvement in how we deliver care in America--not without flaws, but steady progression on the path ahead.

Consumer Focused

We have discussed many patient-centric issues throughout this book and underlying points noted for the baby boomers, Generation X and Y is the broader notion of consumerism in its influence on healthcare over the past decade and for the future. Health insurance changes, new technologies, and care delivery system changes have impacted consumers from the perspective of patient outcomes, safety, satisfaction, and financial burdens.

The need to meet consumer demand in healthcare services is a major driving influence for many of the changes seen in healthcare today. First, the growth and expansion of retail clinics and urgent care clinics has provided a new care delivery setting that meets the needs of added convenience and access to limited scope primary care and emergency care services for consumers and is expected to continue growing for the foreseeable future.[31] Second, the importance of EMRs was discussed in Chapter 4, but for the consumer to have direct access to their digitized health record the development of personal health records (PHR) has provided one such path to enable this capability.

A third issue that has been mentioned is that of telemedicine services. These types of services are improving accessibility to services for consumers through the use of telemedicine technologies and providing new channels for communications between patients, physicians and care provider teams. This is especially helpful in rural communities where access to specialists may be limited. In fact, in May 2011, CMS passed a final rule that streamlined physician and practitioners credentialing for those that provide telemedicine services.[32] For consumers in areas where critical access hospitals (CAH) are their nearest locations to receive medical care, this regulatory change offers an example where lightening regulatory burdens can result in opportunities to expand services that improve patient satisfaction and outcomes for consumers in geographic areas where access to care is limited.

These are but a few additional examples of consumer focus on issues in healthcare today. In the conclusion of *Consumer-centric Healthcare: Opportunities and Challenges for Providers*, Konschak and Jarrell summarized the importance of many of these issues along with the importance of consumers driving the future of healthcare,

Consumers needs and demands will largely dictate which healthcare providers flourish. Effective, forward-thinking leadership is vital.[33]

In Conclusion

We have covered six major initiatives, each of which is worthy of its own book––and many books have been written about each topic over the years. As the U.S. healthcare system and society advance, progress will continue in each of these areas. The IOM discussed the need for system redesign in 2001,[34] and great strides have been made already since then, but much work remains to be done.

Innovations can emerge from efforts both large and small by individuals and organizations. Philanthropic initiatives channel funds into *socially innovative* programs that help us take steps––or at times quantum leaps––to improve the quality of life for the next generation. They tackle the complex issues and challenges requiring an influx of resources that few can provide. Existing challenges in which social innovations will support the advancement of progress include:

- Advanced care for the indigent;

- Eradication of type 2 diabetes through continued improvement in public health and consumer education initiatives;

- Continued improvement of the nation's safety net beyond enactment of the ACA.

In the future as they have been in the past, social innovations in healthcare may be needed to improve sustainability as well as support global social responsibility and citizenship. The needs of the baby boomer generation, Generation X, and Generation Y must also be met while overcoming the systemic challenges of the baby boomer generation. As we reduce the cost, and improve the quality and accessibility of care, new resources can emerge to address the full spectrum of challenges.

Your Next Steps in transforming healthcare involves these initiatives and others to change the way we deliver and pay for healthcare. Actions are taking place across the country and new discoveries arrive daily. To change the U.S. healthcare system we must continue to welcome new ideas and seek opportunities to:

↓ *Test the ideas*

↓ *Separate the good from the bad*

↓ *Appreciate failures and learn from the mistakes*

↓ *Advance the great ideas and get them to market*

Each of us has a chance to contribute. We can choose to be bystanders or to participate in the unfolding.

Now what are your next steps?

We may each have a unique path in life, but coming together to help improve the system for the next generation will make a difference for those around you, in your communities, and throughout our nation.

"Faith is taking the first step even when you don't see the whole staircase."

Martin Luther King, Jr. (1929–1968)
American Clergyman and Civil Rights Leader

30 Porter ME and Teisberg EO. Principles of Value-Based Competition. In: *Redefining Health Care. Creating Value-Based Competition on Results*. Boston, MA: Harvard Business School Publishing, 2006, p. 98.

31 Herrick D. *Retail Clinics: Convenient and Affordable Care*. National Center for Policy Analysis. Brief Analysis 686, January 24, 2010. Accessed online October 28, 2011 at http://www.ncpa.org/pub/ba686.

32 Fed. Reg. vol. 76, no. 87, May 5, 2011. Medicare and Medicaid Programs: Changes Affecting Hospital Conditions of Participation: Telemedicine Credentialing and Privileging. I. Background, p. 25550.

33 Konschak C, Jarrell L. Vision for the Future, In: *Consumer-centric Healthcare: Opportunities and Challenges for Providers*. Chicago, IL: Healthcare Administration Press, 2010, p. 191.

34 Institute of Medicine, Committee on Quality of Health Care in America. Building Organizational Supports for Change. In: *Crossing the Quality Chasm: A New Health System for the 21st Century*. Washington, DC: National Academies Press, 2001, pp. 117–18.

Bibliography

Ash JS, Sittig DF, Poon EG, et al. The extent and importance of unintended consequences related to computerized provider order entry. *J Am Med Infom Assoc.* 2007;14(4):415-423.

Campbell EM, Sittig DF, Ash JS, Guappone KP, Dykstra RH. Types of unintended consequences related to computerized provider order entry. *J Am Med Inform Assoc.* 2006;13(5):547-56.

Christensen, CM., Grossman JH., and Hwang J. *The Innovator's Prescription. A Disruptive Solution for Health Care.* New York, NY: McGraw-Hill, 2009.

DeNavas-Walt, Carmen, Bernadette D. Proctor, and Jessica C. Smith, U.S. Census Bureau, Current Population Reports, P60-239. *Income, Poverty, and Health Insurance Coverage in the United States: 2010*, U.S. Washington, DC: Government Printing Office, 2011.

Fisher ES, McClellan MB, Bertko J, et. al. Fostering accountable health care: moving forward in Medicare. *Health Aff (Millwood).* 2009;28(2):w219-w231.

Flareau B, Yale K, Bohn JM, Konschak C. *Clinical Integration: A Roadmap to Accountable Care.* Virginia Beach: Convurgent Publishing, 2011.

Herrick D. *Retail Clinics: Convenient and Affordable Care.* National Center for Policy Analysis. Brief Analysis 686, January 24, 2010.

Huston L and Sakkab N. Connect and Develop: Inside Procter & Gamble's New Model for Innovation. *Harvard Business Review*, 84 (March 2006):58-66.

Iglehart JK. Defining Essential Health Benefits — The View from the IOM Committee. *New England Journal of Medicine* 365 (October 20, 2011):1461–1463.

Institute of Medicine, Committee on Patient Safety and Health Information Technology. *Health IT and Patient Safety: Building Safer Systems for Better Care*. Washington, DC: The National Academies Press, 2012 (pre-publication copy).

Institute of Medicine, Committee on Quality of Health Care in America. *Crossing the Quality Chasm: A New Health System for the 21st Century*. Washington, DC: National Academies Press, 2001.

Institute of Medicine, Committee on Quality of Health Care in America. Executive Summary. In: *To Err Is Human.* Washington, DC: National Academies Press, 2000.

Kaiser Family Foundation and Health Education & Research Trust. Section One: Cost of Health Insurance. In: *Employer Health Benefits, 2011 Annual Survey.* Menlo Park, CA: Henry J. Kaiser Foundation, 2011.

Konschak C, Jarrell L. *Consumer-centric Healthcare: Opportunities and Challenges for Providers.* Chicago, IL: Healthcare Administration Press, 2010.

Koppel R, Metlay JP, Cohen A, et al. Role of Computerized Physician Order Entry Systems in

Facilitating Medication Errors. *JAMA*, 2005;293(1):1197-1203.

Kotter J. and Rathgeber H. *Our Iceberg Is Melting.* New York, NY: St. Martin's Press, 2005.

Medicare Board of Trustees. *2011 Annual Report of the Boards of Trustees of the Federal Hospital Insurance and Federal Supplementary Medical Insurance Trust Funds.*

Porter ME and Teisberg EO. Principles of Value-Based Competition. In: *Redefining Health Care. Creating Value-Based Competition on Results.* Boston, MA: Harvard Business School Publishing, 2006.

Senge P. *The Fifth Discipline. The Art and Practice of the Learning Organization.* New York, NY: Doubleday Currency Publishing, 1990.

Stanford University. (June 2007). Closing the Quality Gap: A Critical Analysis of Quality Improvement Strategies. *AHRQ Technical Review Number 9. Chapter 5. Conceptual Frameworks and Their Application to Evaluating Care Coordination Interventions,* Section 5b. Methodological Approach, Model 2: Donabedian's Quality Framework.

Teitelbaum JB and Wilensky SE. *Essentials of Health Policy and Law.* Sudbury, MA: Jones and Bartlett Publishers, 2007.

Index

L

M

N

O

P

Appendix A: Select Resources on Healthcare Innovation

1. Federal Government- Healthcare

Agency for Healthcare Research and Quality Innovation Exchange
http://www.innovations.ahrq.gov/

Center for Medicare and Medicaid Innovation
http://innovations.cms.gov/

Centers for Medicare and Medicaid Council on Technology and Innovation
https://www.cms.gov/CouncilonTechInnov/

HHSinnovates Program
http://www.hhs.gov/open/initiatives/hhsinnovates/r3index.html

HHS and the Institute of Medicine's Health Data Initiative
http://www.hhs.gov/open/initiatives/hdi/index.html
http://www.iom.edu/Activities/PublicHealth/HealthData.aspx

National Institute of Health's Small Business Innovative Research Grant Program
http://grants.nih.gov/grants/funding/sbir.htm

National Science Foundation's Industry / University Cooperative Research Centers Program (I/UCRC)
http://www.nsf.gov/funding/pgm_summ.jsp?pims_id=5501

National Science Foundation's Partnership for Innovation Program
http://www.nsf.gov/funding/pgm_summ.jsp?pims_id=5261

Veterans Benefits Administration Innovation Initiative
http://www.whitehouse.gov/open/innovations/vaii

2.   Regional Innovation Clusters- Biotechnology

Connect (San Diego, CA)
http://www.connect.org

Maryland Biotechnology Center (Baltimore, MD)
http://marylandbiocenter.org/

Massachusetts Biotechnology Council   (Boston, MA)
http://www.massbio.org

3.   Not-for-Profit Sector

Council for American Medical Innovation
http://americanmedicalinnovation.org

Council on Competitiveness- Regional Innovation Clusters
http://www.compete.org

Kaiser Permanente Garfield Innovation Center
(San Leandro, CA)
http://xnet.kp.org/innovationcenter/

4.   University/Academic Medicine and Biotechnology Innovation Initiatives

Healthcare Innovation Program (Network of the Atlanta Clinical & Translational Science Institute that includes Emory University, Georgia Tech, and Morehouse College)
http://hip.emory.edu

Johns Hopkins Medicine- Center for Innovation in Quality Patient Care (Baltimore, MD)
http://www.hopkinsmedicine.org/innovation_quality_patient_care/
Larta Institute- Network T2 Consortium
(Southern California University Network)
http://www.larta.org/clientsandprograms/universitiesinstitutesandfoundations/networkt2.aspx

Mayo Clinic Center for Innovation (Minneapolis, MN)
http://centerforinnovation.mayo.edu/

Nucleus Innovation- University of Louisville
(Louisville, KY)
http://www.nucleusky.com

Stanford University Program in Healthcare Innovation
(Palo Alto, CA)
http://www.gsb.stanford.edu/phi/

University of California San Diego Global CONNECT
(San Diego, CA)
http://globalconnect.ucsd.edu/

5.   **Integrated Delivery Networks**

Cleveland Clinic (Ohio)
http://www.clevelandclinic.org/innovations/

Geisinger Health System Innovations (Pennsylvania)
http://www.geisinger.org/innovations/index.html

MedStar Health- Institute for Innovation
(Washington, DC)
http://mi2.org/

www.ingramcontent.com/pod-product-compliance
Lightning Source LLC
Chambersburg PA
CBHW022114280326
41933CB00007B/390